The Anti-Cellulite Diet

A Nutritionist's Guide – More than 40 Delicious Recipes that Will Help You Get Rid of Your Cellulite for Good.

By Laura Hails

Contents

Introduction

The food we eat creates the person that we become, eat healthy, nutritious food and you will look radiant, have more energy, sleep more soundly, become more active, lose excess weight and ultimately, achieve more.

There is no miracle cure for cellulite, there are no overnight solutions, magic creams or potions but there is a solution and that solution lies with your diet. Simply put, eat the right diet combined with the right exercise plan and the results can be dramatic.

Scientific studies have proved that by combining the right foods in our diet with a fitness regime that builds muscle as well as burning calories then the appearance of cellulite can be dramatically reduced.

The more variety and colour you add to your diet the more nutritional benefits you will get from it. This book is filled with more than 40 delicious, easy to make recipes, for you to enjoy. The recipes include the foods that you should be consuming more of to help you lose the pounds and lose the cellulite.

Chapter One

Cellulite Explained

What is cellulite

Cellulite is comprised of fat and fluids trapped in pockets of connective tissue beneath the service of the skin which causes the cells to pucker. The thin layer of connective tissue between fat cells starts to thicken and pull together around the fat, causing tiny dimples and irregularities characteristic with cellulite. The fat inside the cells bulges out and the more fat you have the worse the bulging.

What causes cellulite

Cellulite is essentially the result of too much fat and too little muscle. When the underlying muscle becomes too thin and the overlying fat becomes too thick, there is no firm base for the skin, which then takes on the wobbly, irregular appearance we call cellulite.

Failing to do enough exercise has serious consequences. Without regular toning exercise you start to lose muscle after the age of 20. Between the ages of 20 and 30 years the average non-exercise woman loses 5lb of muscle, a further 5lb between the ages of 30 and 40 and a similar amount each decade after that. The result is a loss of strength as well as increase in fat storage.

As you lose muscle, your metabolic rate drops. Muscle burns calories, so the less you have the fewer calories you need. So, as you get older you need fewer calories just to maintain your body weight. For every 5lbs loss of muscle, your metabolic rate drops by 5%.

Age related muscle loss means that you burn fewer calories and store more of them as fat. Even if you continue eating the same amount of food and keeping the same lifestyle, your weight will increase as your body converts the excess calories into stored fat.

For most women this extra fat is stored around the hips and thighs. When an area has too much fat, too little muscle and weak connective tissue, it loses its normal firm appearance and takes on the characteristic wobbly appearance associated with cellulite.

How to fight cellulite

Getting rid of cellulite is not easy and cannot be done overnight. Whilst there are many claims of cellulite cures ranging from diets and pills to creams and treatments scientific studies have shown that the most effective way to get rid of cellulite is a combination of the right diet and the right exercise.

Reducing your calorie intake whilst increasing your daily calorie burn creates a calorie deficit so your body has no choice but to use up its fat stores.

Diet

1 - Eat five or more portions of fruit and vegetables each day

2 - Avoid saturated and processed fats

3 - Eat foods high in fibre and water

4 - Include wholegrains and cereals in your daily diet

5 - Eat more beans and lentils

6 - Eat nuts and seeds regularly

7 - Drink 2 litres of water a day

8 - Avoid refined sugars and flour.

Exercise

The key is to include both strength (toning) training to build muscle as well as cardiovascular (aerobic) exercise to burn fat in your exercise programme. Strength training doesn't necessarily mean lifting heavy weights. It can be toning exercises using your own body weight, light hand-held weights, exercise bands or tubes for resistance.

Don't be afraid of adding strength exercises, as your muscles tone up, they'll become firmer and smaller. As you get older collagen and elastin fibres become less elastic which makes your fat more noticeable. But as you build muscle, the fibres are strengthened, reducing dimples, so the appearance of your cellulite will dramatically improve.

More muscle means more calories burned during activity as well as when resting. Every 1lb of muscle you add through exercise increases your metabolic rate by 30 – 40 calories a day.

Chapter Two
Eat the Rainbow

Antioxidants

Antioxidants come up frequently in discussions about good health and preventing diseases. These powerful substances, which mostly come from the fresh fruits and vegetables we eat, prohibit (and in some cases even prevent), the oxidation of other molecules in the body. The benefits of antioxidants are very important to good health, because if free radicals are left unchallenged, they can cause a wide range of illnesses and chronic diseases.

Antioxidants and Free Radicals

The human body naturally produces free radicals and the antioxidants to counteract their damaging effects. However, in most cases, free radicals far outnumber the naturally occurring antioxidants. In order to maintain the balance, and maximise the benefits of antioxidants a continual supply of external sources of antioxidants are necessary. Antioxidants benefit the body by neutralising and removing the free radicals from the bloodstream.

Different Antioxidants Benefit Different Parts of the Body

There are a wide range of antioxidants found in nature, and because they are so varied, different antioxidants provide benefits to different parts of the body. For example, beta-carotene (and other carotenoids) is very beneficial for healthy eyes, lycopene is beneficial for helping maintain prostate health; flavonoids are especially beneficial in maintaining a healthy heart; and proanthocyanins are beneficial for urinary tract health.

Antioxidants and Skin Health Benefits

When skin is exposed to high levels of ultraviolet light, photo-oxidative damage is induced by the formation of different types of reactive species of oxygen, including singlet oxygen, superoxide radicals, and peroxide radicals. These forms of reactive oxygen damage cellular lipids, proteins, and DNA, and they are considered to be the primary contributors to erythema (sunburn), premature aging of the skin, photo dermatoses, and skin cancers.

Antioxidants and Immune System Support

Singlet oxygen can compromise the immune system, because it has the ability to catalyze production of free radicals. Astaxanthin and Spirulina have been shown to enhance both the non-specific and specific immune system, and to protect cell membranes and cellular DNA from mutation. Astaxanthin is the single most powerful quencher of singlet oxygen, and is up to ten times stronger than other carotenoids (including beta-carotene), and up to 500 times stronger than alpha tocopherol (Vitamin E), while Spirulina has a variety of antioxidants and other substances that are beneficial in boosting immunity.

Additional Ways Antioxidants Help Benefit our Health

Increasing one's antioxidant intake is essential for optimum health, especially in today's polluted world. Because the body just can't keep up with antioxidant production, a good amount of these vitamins, minerals, phytochemicals, and enzymes must come from our daily diet. Boosting your antioxidant intake can help provide added protection for the body against heart problems, eye problems, memory problems, mood disorders and immune system problems.

Top Antioxidant – rich Fruit and Vegetables.

Blackberries, blueberries, broccoli, Brussel sprouts, Curly kale, garlic, plums, prunes, raisins, raspberries, red peppers, spinach and strawberries.

Plant Nutrients -

The more variety and colour you eat the more nutrients you will consume and the more benefit you will get from your diet.

According to a recent National Diet and Nutrition Survey many of our diets - adults and children - are lacking in vitamin A and D, selenium and zinc and many women are lacking calcium and iron.

Fruit and vegetables are considered so good for us that nutritionists suggest that the recommended government 5 a day should be our bare minimum. But the truth is that most people aren't even eating 5 a day. Fruit and vegetables provide a huge variety of vitamins, minerals and fibre and if you are missing out on eating them you will leave a big gap in the nutrients you consume.

The best way to get the most from your food is variety. Many people get stuck in a rut, eating the same food day in and day out with little or no variety. In order to stay healthy, the body needs over 40 different vitamins and minerals a day so sticking to the same foods will hugely reduce your intake.

Introducing new and different foods to your weekly shop will not only keep your food exciting but your body will reap the rewards.

Whilst some foods have significant health benefits it is important to remember that no one individual food can treat, prevent or cure health problems, the key is to eat all foods as part of a balanced diet.

Include fruit and vegetables from the five colour groups, red, orange, yellow, green and purple. Different coloured fruit and vegetables contain different nutrients, combining them is the best way to ensure you get all you need.

Many of the naturally occurring chemicals responsible for giving fruit and veg their bright colours actually help keep us healthy and free from disease. Fruit and vegetables contain hundreds of colourful phytochemicals that act as antioxidants.

Antioxidant-rich fruit and vegetables can help to protect against heart disease, cancer, and premature aging.

Red–

Many red foods contain high levels of vitamin C. They contain high levels of anthocyanins which are linked to being effective in fighting cancer, bacterial infections and neurological diseases.

Red fruit and vegetables to include in your diet

are raspberries, cranberries, strawberries, cherries, pomegranate, apples, rhubarb, red peppers, tomatoes and watermelon.

Orange

Orange fruit and vegetables are high in carotenoids, crucial for maintaining a good immune system and supporting cell repair and healthy vision.

Orange fruit and vegetables to include in your diet are Carrots, oranges, squashes, sweet potatoes, mangoes, peaches, nectarines, pumpkins, swede and peppers.

Yellow

Yellow fruit and vegetables contain large amounts of bioflavonoids, which fight infection and reduce inflammation.

Yellow fruit and vegetables to introduce into your diet – corn, pineapple, peppers and squashes.

Green

Green fruit and vegetables contain nutrients including lutein, lycopene, folic acid, zeaxanthin and glycosylates all of which are associated with helping to prevent cancer.

Green fruit and vegetables to include in your diet

- asparagus, avocado, rocket, spinach, lettuce, watercress, cucumber, broccoli, Brussels sprouts, leafy cabbage, spring greens, beans, peas, sugar snap peas, mange tout, cress, courgette, peppers, spring onions, leeks, apples, grapes and kiwi fruit.

Purple/blue

Purple and blue fruit and vegetables are high in antioxidants which promote healthy blood and are believed to have antiaging properties.

Purple and blue fruit and vegetables to include in your diet are blackberries, blueberries, grapes, blackcurrants, plums, red cabbage, prunes, red onions, olives, purple sprouting broccoli, beetroot and aubergine.

Chapter Three

Rules for Healthy Living.

Cook from scratch

Take responsibility for what you are eating by knowing exactly what is in your food. Cooking from scratch doesn't have to be complicated or time consuming. look for quick, simple recipes, the fewer the ingredients the quicker the dish, and use good quality ingredients to maximise nutrition. Plan ahead and know what you are going to cook and adapt your menu to the time you have. The recipes in this plan will help you do just that.

Read the labels

Food labels are a reliable, accurate source of valuable nutritional information. Use the labels on the foods you buy to ensure that you are consuming what you think you are consuming. Ingredients are listed in descending order by weight and include any colour, additives, preservatives and, nutrients, fats or sugar that have been added to the product.

Whatever appears first on the list is the largest ingredient. Foods with high levels of sugar, salt or saturated fats at the top of the list should be avoided.

Know your Sugar

Sugar comes in many forms with many different names, but it is all the same and has the same effect on the body. Products with sugar listed at the top of its ingredients list is more than likely high in sugar. The following are all sugars – brown sugar, cane juice lactose, maltose, raw cane sugar, raw sugar, sucrose sugar, invert sugar, glucose, fructose, dextrose, corn syrup, corn sweetener.

Consider naturally sweet alternatives such as raw honey or maple syrup or add fruit such as apples, apricots and berries. Carrot or apple juice makes a great base for vegetable juices as they add sweetness.

Know Your Fats

Good fats or "essential fatty acids" as they are known come from nuts and seeds, fish and avocados, they are important for a healthy, balanced diet. These can also be added to your cooking by using them as oils such as sunflower and pumpkin seed oil, macadamia, coconut, walnut, hazelnut and olive oils are all beneficial fats that support nerve function, mental alertness, concentration and memory.

Bad fats or saturated / trans fats are known to raise levels of cholesterol and increase the risk of heart disease. These are found mainly in animal produce and dairy products they are in butter, lard, margarine, cooking fats, chocolate, biscuits, cakes, savoury snacks and processed foods.

Read the label and avoid anything that says it contains "hydrogenated" or "partially hydrogenated oils"

Add colour

The more colour in your diet the more goodness you will consume. Each colour of fruit and vegetables contains different and important antioxidants. Antioxidants are part of a well- balanced, healthy diet, they will keep you well throughout the winter months by helping your immune system to kill harmful bacteria and infections and they will keep your skin and hair looking good and give you vitality. Vitamins A, C and E are all found in fresh fruit and vegetables and are all antioxidants.

Be prepared

Always make a meal plan and a shopping list before shopping. Consider the week ahead in advance. Think about foods that you love and how you can introduce more variety to them. Don't be afraid to find recipes and tweak them to suit your own tastes you may discover something wonderful.

Consider days that you might be home late or have more work to do than normal and make those evening meals simple and quick or even prepare them at the weekend, or when you have more time, and freeze them so that they are at hand when you need a quick meal. Making your own microwave meals doesn't need to be either complicated or time consuming – it just needs planning. Consider, omelets, stir fries or salads with fresh or tinned fish.

Stay Hydrated

Dehydration can, falsely, make you think that you are hungry. Your brain can confuse thirst with hunger. Before reaching for a biscuit or sweets make a conscious effort to have a glass of water and then decide whether you were hungry or thirsty. If you really are hungry consider what you are reaching for.

Healthy Snacking.

Snacking between meals is a good thing. As long as you make the right choices, healthy snacking keeps your blood sugars level and increases your energy. Snacking keeps your brain active meaning that you can concentrate and remain focused throughout the day and on into the evening.

If you enjoy your snacks, aim for fruit, plain or unsweetened Greek-style yogurt, celery sticks, carrots or nuts and seeds.

Not Just 5 a Day

We all know that 5 portions of fruit and vegetables a day is the recommended amount. Given the nutritional value in fruit and vegetables and the health benefits of them 5 portions should be your absolute minimum and whilst meal planning you should be looking at ways of increasing your consumption wherever you can.

Try adding fruit to your breakfast cereal or drinking a smoothie instead of a cup of tea for breakfast, be more adventurous with your salads, replace your lunchtime sandwich and crisps with a salad and add vegetables to your pasta sauces, stews and soups and before you know it you will have increased your intake of fruit and veg without even noticing.

Flavour Your Food with Herbs and Spices.

Spices have been found to inhibit the formation of prostaglandins – the hormones that trigger inflammatory reactions. Reduce your use of salt and increase your use of herbs and mild spices to flavour your food instead. Use - cloves, cinnamon, turmeric, rosemary, ginger, sage, and thyme all of which are known for their anti-inflammatory properties.

Scientists in India have found that curcumin, the primary active ingredient of turmeric, has anti – depressant qualities that were found to be at least as effective as certain medications in the treatment of depression – but without the negative side effects.

Refined V Unrefined

Always choose unrefined ingredients over refined ones.

Unrefined foods contain more natural nutrients because they have not been stripped of their vitamins and minerals in the refining process.

Fibre

People who eat a lot of refined foods and skip the fruit and vegetables are missing out on fibre. A lack of fibre in the diet leads to digestive problems and blood sugar imbalances. Fibre is the indigestible portion of grains, vegetables and fruit it is used by the body to improve intestinal function, helps to grow healthy bacteria in the gut and helps prevent disease by removing waste products and toxins from the body. Drop the white bread, pasta and rice and increase fruit, vegetables and whole grains wherever possible.

Eat at least 25 grams of fibre every day. A fibre-rich diet helps reduce inflammation by supplying the body with anti-inflammatory phytonutrients found in fruits, vegetables, and other whole foods. The best sources of fibre are whole grains, such as barley and oatmeal; vegetables such as peas, Brussel sprouts, parsnips and spinach, and fruit such as apples, bananas, oranges, strawberries and raspberries.

Recipes

Apples.

Apples are low in calories and high in fibre. They are full of antioxidants which help flush out toxins from the body as well as containing pectin which is a gel forming fibre that helps to detox the digestive tract, helping to break down cellulite. –

Apple Coleslaw

Serves 4

Ingredients
½ a small red cabbage
2 crisp, hard apples – cored and sliced
4 / 5 strips of sundried tomatoes in oil – drained and chopped
4 salad onions – finely chopped
2 tbsp. mixed seeds
50g feta cheese
1 lime – juice
2 tbsp extra virgin olive oil
50g raisins
2 tbsp pine nuts

. Finely slice the cabbage and place in a large serving bowl.

. Stir in the chopped apples, sundried tomatoes, salad onions, mixed seeds and raisins.

. whisk the lime juice and olive oil together and pour over the salad.

. Crumble over the feta and sprinkle with the pine nuts.

Apple and Feta Waldorf salad

Serves 4

Ingredients
100g walnuts

5 tbsp mayonnaise

5 tbsp. greek yoghurt

1 lemon – juice

150g Feta cheese

2 firm apples

4 celery stalks – finely sliced

2 large handfuls watercress.

. Heat the oven to 180C / gas 4.

. Spread the walnuts on a baking tray and roast for 10 – 12 minutes until just turning golden brown.

. Place the mayonnaise, Greek yogurt and lemon juice in a blender with 1/3 of the feta and blend until smooth.

.

Add the apples, celery and most of the walnuts to the dressing and stir until everything is coated. Crumble the remaining feta and stir through the mixture.

. Place the watercress onto a serving plate spoon on the walnut and feta mix and top with the rest of the walnuts.

Apricots

Apricots are rich in fibre and high in vitamins A and C as well as containing lycopene which helps to reduce water retention and stimulate circulation both of which can help fight cellulite.

Apricot Breakfast Bars

Makes – 16 bars

Ingredients
1 cup almonds

1 cup cashews

12 dried apricots – roughly chopped

½ cup raisins

½ cup mixed seeds

½ cup chocolate chips

½ honey

.Heat the oven to 180C and line a square 20cm tin with parchment paper

. Place the almonds, cashews, seeds and apricots into a blender and blend until roughly chopped.

. Pour the mix into a mixing bowl and add the raisins, and chocolate chips, pour over the honey and stir until completely combined.

Pour the mixture into the lined tin and press firmly down.

. Place in the oven for 20 – 25 minutes. Leave to cool and the refrigerate for an hour before turning out and cutting into 16 bars.

Asparagus

Asparagus is high in anti-inflammatory properties which are known to reduce bloating. It is also low in calories making it perfect for those looking to reduce their weight. Asparagus is also known to stimulate the bloods circulation which helps to flush out toxins that can lead to cellulite.

Asparagus and Pea Risotto
Serves: - 4

Ingredients: -
3 tbsp. olive oil
2 shallots – finely chopped
1 garlic clove – crushed
300g risotto rice
1 ltre. Hot vegetable stock
400g asparagus – trimmed
100g frozen peas
75ml dry white wine
85g parmesan shavings

Heat the olive oil in a large pan, add the shallots and cook for about 5 minutes until soft. Add the rice and the garlic and stir to coat the rice in the oil. Pour in the wine and stir until it has been absorbed.

Ladle a spoon of stock into the rice, stirring constantly until all the liquid has been absorbed. Repeat the process until you are left with about 200ml of stock – approximately 15 - 20 minutes.

Add the asparagus and peas and the remaining 200ml of stock and simmer until all the liquid has been absorbed, season and sprinkle over the parmesan shavings.

Bananas

Bananas are known for being a great energy source as well as being high in zinc which helps to improve the skin. The potassium found in bananas helps to boost blood flow which can help to prevent cellulite.

Banana and Blueberry Crush
Serves: - 2

Ingredients: -
1 banana – peeled
300ml – almond milk
150g frozen blueberries
A large handful of oats

Place the oats in a jug or bowl, cover with the almond milk and set aside for 10 minutes.
Place the blueberries into a blender along with ½ the almond milk and blend. Add the banana and the remaining milk and blend again.

Beans

Aduki beans, borlotti beans, cannelloni beans, Chickpeas, haricot beans, Kidney beans and lentils are high in protein and fibre they contain iron, potassium, magnesium as well as B vitamins.

Beans help to regulate the appetite, lower cholesterol, control blood pressure and help you lose weight which can help to get rid of cellulite. Beans provide a lot of bulk without a lot of calories which fills you up and keeps you satisfied for longer.

Spring Greens and Cannellini Bean Soup
Serves: - 6

Ingredients: -
2 tbsp. olive oil
3 celery sticks – finely chopped
1 red onion – chopped
2 carrots – chopped
1 garlic clove – crushed
2 tins 400g chopped tomatoes
1 x 400g tin cannellini beans – drained and rinsed
100g shredded spring greens
800ml vegetable stock

Small bunch of basil

Heat the oil in a large saucepan, add the celery, onion, carrots and garlic and cook on a low heat for 20 minutes until soft.
Add the tomatoes and cook for a further 20 minutes.
Add the beans and cook for a further 10 minutes before adding the stock. Bring the soup to the boil and simmer for 5 minutes.
Add the shredded spring greens and simmer for a further 5 minutes until everything is tender. Season before serving.

Broad Bean Dip

Serves: - 4

Ingredients: -

350g baby broad beans – podded and skinned

1 shallot – finely chopped

100g ricotta

2 tbsp. flat leaf parsley – chopped

1 tbsp. mint – chopped

2 tbsp. extra virgin olive oil

Place the beans into a blender and blend until coarse, add the shallot, ricotta, herbs and 1 tbsp. of the olive oil and blend briefly.

Add the rest of the oil, season and blend again.

<u>*Cannellini and Vegetable Soup*</u>

Serves – 4

Ingredients

2 tbsp Olive oil

1 medium red onion – peeled and sliced

2 medium carrots – peeled and sliced

2 medium leeks – sliced

400g cannellini beans, drained and rinsed

800ml vegetable stock

50g quinoa.

. Heat the oil in a pan and fry the onions, leeks and carrots for 3 – 4 minutes.

.Add the beans, stock and quinoa and bring to the boil, cover and simmer until the vegetables and quinoa are tender.

Beetroot

This beautifully coloured root vegetable contains lycopene which helps stimulate circulation as well as reduce water retention. Beetroots also contain potassium which helps boost blood flow, vitamin E which is essential for healthy skin and vitamin A which boosts collagen in the skin.

Beetroot Pesto

Serves 4

Ingredients: -

1 large roasted beetroot

1 tbsp. flat leaf parsley – chopped

½ lemon – juice and zest

Handful wild rocket

1 garlic clove – crushed

2 tbsp. extra virgin olive oil

Handful toasted hazelnuts

2 tsp. capers

1 tbsp. crème fraiche

Place all the ingredients into a blender and blend until a smooth paste is formed. If you want a looser consistency add more oil.

Beetroot and Lentil Salad

Serves: - 2

Ingredients: -

2 tbsp. virgin olive oil

1 red onion – halved and sliced

250g cooked lentils (tin or packet)

200g small cooked beetroots – cut into wedges

1 tbsp. sherry vinegar

½ large pack rocket

Heat 1 tbsp. olive oil in a pan and cook the onion for a few minutes until starting to colour.

Tip the lentils into the pan, add the beetroot wedges, vinegar, remaining oil, a little seasoning and a tbsp. of water. Cover the pan and heat for a couple of minutes until it has warmed through.

Spoon onto a serving plate, stir through the rocket and serve.

Beetroot and Sugar Snap Pea Salad

Serves: - 6

Ingredients: -

100g beetroot – peeled, trimmed and cut into wedges

3 tbsp. extra virgin olive oil

Zest ½ orange

500g sugar snap peas – trimmed

2 thyme sprigs

1 tbsp. sherry vinegar

½ shallot – finely chopped

Heat the oven to 180C / gas 4,

Mix together the oil and ½ the orange zest and toss the prepared beetroot in it, then place them on a large sheet of tin foil, season and cook for 45 minutes until tender. Leave to cool.

Steam the sugar snap peas for 1 – 2 minutes until tender. Drain, cool under the cold tap and drain again.

Strip the leaves from the thyme, whisk with the remaining oil, vinegar and chopped shallot. Place the beetroot wedges and peas on a serving plate, stir through the vinegar dressing and sprinkle over the remaining orange zest.

Cranberry and Beetroot Red Cabbage

Serves: - 6

Ingredients: -

1 tbsp. olive oil

4 shallots – finely chopped

2 tbsp. maple syrup

½ tsp. mixed spice

½ red cabbage (650g) – thinly sliced

Zest and juice 1 orange

150ml port

Large sprig thyme

Splash red wine vinegar

200g cranberries

3 medium cooked beetroots – sliced

Flat leaf parsley – to decorate

Heat the oil in a large, shallow pan and gently fry the onions for 5 minutes until soft. Add the maple syrup and spice and cook for a further 2 minutes.

Stir in the cabbage and coat it in the spices. Add the zest and juice of the orange, the port, thyme leaves and red wine vinegar along with 100ml of water. Stir through, cover and cook over a low heat for 1 hour until tender.

Add the cranberries for the last 20 minutes of cooking time and the beetroot for the last 5 minutes to heat through. Decorate with the chopped parsley before serving.

Berries

Berries are a rich source of toxin fighting antioxidants. Regularly eating raspberries, blackberries, strawberries, cranberries and blueberries is a good way of flushing toxins from the body.

Blueberry Smoothie

Makes 1 Glass

Ingredients: -

75g blueberries

1 small banana – peeled and cut into chunks

2 tbsp. fromage frais

2 tbsp. maple syrup

75ml milk

Place all the ingredients into a blender and blend until smooth.

Wake Me Up Smoothie

Serves – 2

Ingredients: -

200g raspberries

250g plain live bio-yoghurt

50g porridge oats

3 tbsp. maple syrup

2 sprigs of mint.

Place all the ingredients into a blender and blend until smooth.

Broccoli

Broccoli is high in nutritional value. Each floret contains high levels of beauty boosting vitamins and minerals as well as being low in calories.

Broccoli also contains Alpha lipoic which is a naturally occurring substance that prevents collagen from hardening in the body which results in cellulite.

Broccoli with Anchovies and Garlic

Serves: - 4

Ingredients: -

500g purple sprouting broccoli

Olive oil

2 cloves garlic – peeled and crushed

5 anchovy fillets

Pinch of chilli flakes

Juice of ½ a lime

Trim the broccoli and steam over boiling water until tender – for about 4 minutes. Drain, reserving a little of the water from the steamer.

Heat a little oil in a pan, add the garlic, anchovies and chilli flakes and stir until the anchovies have melted.

Add the broccoli, a little of the reserved water, cover and cook for about 1 minute, until soft. Add lemon juice and a little seasoning.

Tenderstem Broccoli with Cream Cheese and Rosemary

Serves: - 6

Ingredients: -

2 tbsp. olive oil

50g cream cheese

1 garlic clove – peeled and crushed

2 small pinches of dried chilli flakes

2 small rosemary sprigs – leaves finely chopped

Small squeeze of Lime juice

500g tenderstem broccoli

Place the cream cheese, garlic, chilli, chopped rosemary leaves, and a small squeeze of lime juice into a blender and blend. Roll into a ball and chill.

Cook the broccoli in a steamer for about 5 minutes until tender, drain and place on a serving plate. Roughly break the cream cheese into small pieces and sprinkle over the broccoli.

Broccoli, Pea and Ricotta Frittata

Serves: - 4

Ingredients: -

125g broccoli florets

260g spinach

3 tbsp. ricotta

1 garlic clove – peeled and crushed

1 tbsp. olive oil

1 onion – finely chopped

160g frozen peas

6 eggs – beaten

Heat the oven to 200C / gas 6.

Place the spinach into a colander and pour boiling water over it to wilt it. Rinse under cold water to cool and then squeeze out the liquid and chop.

Steam the broccoli for 4 – 5 minutes until just tender, drain and set aside.

Mix the ricotta and garlic together and season.

Purple Sprouting Broccoli and Wild Rice

Serves: -2

Ingredients: -

2 tbsp. olive oil

2 cloves garlic – crushed

150g wild rice

230g purple sprouting broccoli

Lemon zest

100g feta cheese

Large handful mixed seeds

Cook the wild rice according to the packet instructions. Trim the broccoli and add it to the wild rice two minutes before the rice is finished cooking. Drain.

Heat the oil and garlic in a large frying pan for about 2 minutes before adding the rice and broccoli. Toss the oil through the rice, season and add the lemon zest.

Place on a serving plate and crumble over the feta and sprinkle with the mixed seeds.

Cucumber

Cucumber is a diuretic food, which can help relieve water retention and flush out toxins from the body. A build-up of fluid in the body can trigger the formation of cellulite.

Cucumber and Elderflower Salad

Serves 4

Ingredients: -
1 cucumber – sliced finely
1 tsp. sugar
1 tsp. salt
1 tbsp. white wine vinegar
250ml water
1 tbsp. elderflower syrup
1 tbsp. olive oil
Mixed fresh herbs of your choice - chopped

Add the sugar, salt and vinegar to the water, place the cucumber slices to the mixture and steep for a couple of hours. Drain thoroughly and pat dry.

Mix the elderflower syrup and olive oil together, toss the cucumber in it and gently stir through the chopped mixed herbs.

If elderflowers are in season – sprinkle with a handful of freshly picked flowers.

Mackerel with Tomatoes and Cucumber Salsa Verde

Serves 4

Ingredients: -

2 anchovy fillets in oil – drained

½ garlic clove – crushed

1 tsp. Dijon mustard

14g mint leaves – chopped

14g – flat leaf parsley – chopped

14g basil – chopped

100ml olive oil

¼ cucumber – peeled and diced

4 x 200g mackerel fillets

270g cherry tomatoes

1 lemon

Heat the oven to 220C/ gas 7. Place the anchovies, garlic, mustard and chopped herbs to a blender and blend, whilst the motor is running drizzle in 6 tbsp. olive oil until the paste is blended. Stir in the cucumber and season to taste.

Brush the fish with a little oil and season. Place the fish in a lightly oiled baking tray along with the tomatoes bake for 8 – 10 minutes until the fish is cooked through.

Squeeze over a little lemon juice and serve with the salsa verde.

Dandelion Tea

Dandelion, like nettles, with its diuretic properties is a liver tonic. Dandelion helps rid the body of toxins and flush out excess fluids. Dandelion is a powerful antioxidant, containing vitamins A, C, D and E, zinc, iron and potassium.

Fennel

Fennel aids digestion, reduces inflammation and helps to flush out the excess fluid and toxins that can lead to cellulite. Fennel is also excellent for maintaining healthy hair and skin.

Fennel and Roast Tomato Lasagne

Serves: - 4

Ingredients: -

3 fennel bulbs – thinly sliced

3 tbsp. extra virgin olive oil

800g vine tomatoes

2 tbsp. balsamic vinegar

100ml natural yoghurt

50ml crème fraiche

150g hard cheese - grated

250g whole wheat lasagne sheets.

Heat the oven to 180C/ gas 4.

Place the fennel into a large roasting tray, season and drizzle with 2 tbsp. of the oil.

Leaving the tomatoes on the vine, place them in a separate tray, season and drizzle with the remaining oil and the balsamic vinegar. Roast both vegetables for 30 minutes.

Mix ½ the grated cheese, yoghurt and crème fraiche together and stir it through the fennel and return it to the oven for a further 10 minutes.

To assemble: -

Spoon a third of the fennel onto the bottom of an ovenproof dish, place a third of the tomatoes and top with a layer of lasagne sheets. Repeat.

Spoon over the final third of fennel, topped with the remaining tomatoes, sprinkle over the rest of the cheese and bake for 45 minutes until golden.

Garlic

Garlic helps lower cholesterol and boosts the immune system which not only helps to improve the body's overall health but also aids the blood circulation which helps to flush out toxins and fight cellulite.

Pasta with Wild Garlic Sauce
Serves 2

Ingredients: -
2 tbsp. olive oil
2 shallot finely chopped
120g wild garlic – chopped
250ml tomato passata
A splash of sherry vinegar
150g dried tagliatelle
Parmesan shavings

Heat the olive oil in a frying pan over a medium heat, add the shallots and gently fry for 2 minutes, add the wild garlic and cook for a further 5 – 7 minutes, until softened.
Add the passata and vinegar, season, reduce the heat and leave to simmer for a further 10 minutes.

Cook the tagliatelle as per the packed instructions, drain and add to the pan, stir through and serve with parmesan shavings.

Wild garlic Soup

Serves 4

Ingredients: -
2 tbsp. olive oil
270g potatoes – peeled and chopped
240g red onions – peeled and chopped
180g wild garlic – chopped
500ml vegetable stock
Crème fraiche – to serve.

Heat the olive oil in a large saucepan and add the onions and potatoes and season, saute for about five minutes.
Add the garlic and continue to cook for a further 5 minutes until the garlic is tender. Pour in the stock, cover and simmer for 40 minutes.
Pour into a blender and blend until smooth, return to the pan, season and reheat.
Spoon over the crème fraiche and serve.

Lemons

Lemons can aid the rebalancing of the body's acid-alkali keeping it at a steady PH, meaning that your body is better able to support healthy bacteria and assist the removal of toxins which can lead to cellulite.

Tomato, Wild Rice and Roasted Lemon Salad

Serves 4

Ingredients: -

3 tbsp. olive oil

½ tsp. brown sugar

400g cherry tomatoes – halved

14g flat leaf parsley

28g mint

1 pomegranate – seeds removed

1 ½ tbsp. balsamic vinegar

½ small red onion – finely sliced

100g mixed wild rice

2 medium lemons – halved lengthways and cut width ways into 2mm slices.

Heat the oven to 200C / gas 6

Bring a small pan of water to the boil and blanch the lemon slices for 2 minutes, then place them in a bowl and pour over 1 tbsp. oil and ½ tsp. of sugar and ½ tsp. of salt.

Place the lemons onto a baking tray and bake for 20 minutes. Cook the wild rice as per the packet instructions, drain and set aside.

Place the rest of the ingredients in a bowl, add the cooked wild rice and stir through the remaining oil, add the baked lemon slices and season with a little salt and pepper before serving.

Lemon and Roasted Tomatoes

Serves: - 2

Ingredients: -

200g mozzarella

¼ lemon

3 garlic cloves – crushed

270g cherry vine tomatoes

3 tbsp. olive oil

Small handful basil leaves

Heat the oven to 160C/ gas mark 2.

Cut the lemon in to thin slices, toss in a roasting tray along with the tomatoes, garlic and olive oil. Season and roast for 20 minutes.

Tear the mozzarella into bite size pieces and place on a serving plate, lay the tomatoes on top and pour over the lemon and juices.

Scatter over the roughly torn basil leaves.

Live Bio Yoghurt

Live bio yoghurt is full of probiotics and in terms of aiding weight loss it is considered a superfood. Yoghurt is now known to have a significant impact on eliminating fat from the body and that includes cellulite.

Raspberry Frozen Yoghurt
Serves: - 6

Ingredients: -
125g raspberries
500g thick, plain, live bio yoghurt
60ml maple syrup
1 tsp. vanilla extract

Place the raspberries, yoghurt, syrup and vanilla extract into a blender and blend. Place in the freezer for 1 hour, stir and replace in the freezer.
Remove from the freezer 1 hour before serving.
If you have an ice cream maker churn for 25 minutes and freeze until firm.

Raspberry Mousse

Serve: - 2

Ingredients: -

200g raspberries

1 tbsp. maple syrup

2 egg whites

150g fat free natural bio yoghurt

3 sheets gelatin sheets

Gently cook the raspberries in a pan with the syrup for 3 – 4 minutes, then sieve, discard the seeds and chill for 10 minutes.

Whisk 2 egg whites until stiff.

Place the yoghurt into a bowl and mix in 100ml of the raspberry mix. Place 3 sheets of gelatin in a large jug, add 1 ½ tbsp. of boiling water and leave to dissolve.

Add the dissolved egg white to the yoghurt mixture, beat in one third of the egg whites, then fold in the remainder.

Pour into serving bowls and chill for 4 – 5 hours.

Decorate with raspberries.

Mango

Mangos are packet with vitamins C and E as well as potassium. Mangos also contain beta-carotene which promotes healthy new cells and boosts the natural elasticity of the skin, creating smoother more evenly textured skin even in cellulite affected areas. The vitamin C in mangos helps to strengthen collagen in the skin.

<u>Caribbean Cream</u>

Serves 4

Ingredients: -

1 Mango – peeled and flesh removed from the stone

400g pineapple – peeled and diced

½ Lime – juice

1 banana – peeled and chopped

150ml almond milk

Place all the ingredients into a blender and blend until smooth and creamy.

Nettles

Nettles are packed with antioxidants. Their diuretic properties help to eliminate the toxins that cause cellulite and relieve water retention.

Nettle Soup

Serves 6

Ingredients: -

4 medium potatoes – peeled and cubed

50g butter

4 shallots – peeled and chopped

2 sticks of celery – chopped

8 wild garlic leaves – torn

450g young nettle tops

3 tbsp. crème fraiche

1litre of vegetable stock

Place the potatoes into a pan of salted water, bring to the boil and cook for 15 minutes until tender.

Melt the butter in a large pan and cook the celery, wild garlic and shallots for about ten minutes until soft but not brown.

Using rubber gloves discard any woody/ tough stems from the nettles, wash them and blanch them in boiling water for 2 - 3 minutes.

Add the stock, potatoes and blanched nettles to the shallots, simmer for 5 – 10 minutes until the nettles tender. Place in a blender and blend until smooth. Return to the pan.

Stir in the crème fraiche, season to taste and re heat before serving.

Nuts

Walnuts, almonds, brazils, cashews, hazelnuts, macadamia, peanuts, pine nuts, pistachios and walnuts are all high sources of fibre, and protein. They contain vitamins B and E, potassium and magnesium.

Snacking on nuts will help curb hunger, feed your skin and lower your cholesterol and help control blood pressure. Nuts help you lose weight.

Mushroom and Walnut Pesto
Serves 4

Ingredients: -
320g closed cap mushrooms – fried in 1 tbsp. olive oil

2 garlic cloves – crushed

2 tbsp. walnut oil

½ tsp. dried rosemary

½ lemon – juice

Handful Flat leaf parsley – chopped

Handful walnuts

Place all of the ingredients into a blender and blend until the form a loose paste. If you would like a looser consistency all a little more oil.

Oily Fish

Oily fish contain "good fats". Good fats contain fatty acids which can help the body to metabolise fat including cellulite fat. Oily fish include salmon, mackerel, sardines, anchovies and tuna.

Avoid "bad fats" found in processed foods such as biscuits, pastries, cheese and sausages. These fats cause cellulite.

Sardines with Green Beans, Spinach and Potatoes.

Serves 4

Ingredients: -

500g new potatoes

200g green beans

2 tbsp. capers

28g flat leaf parsley – chopped

75g baby spinach leaves

1 garlic clove – crushed

4 spring onions – chopped

4 tbsp. extra virgin olive oil

1 lemon – zest and juice

500g sardines

Boil the potatoes in a pan of salted water for about 15 minutes until tender, add the beans to the last 3 minutes of the potatoes cooking time. Drain and set aside.

Place the capers, parsley, half the spinach leaves, garlic, spring onions and a drizzle of olive oil into a blender and blend, when combined add the zest and juice of the lemon and season. Add more olive oil to loosen it if needed.

Add half the sauce to the potatoes and green beans and toss together and add the remaining spinach leaves.

Rub the sardines with a little olive oil and place on a hot griddle or under a hot grill for 2 – 3 minutes on each side. Place on top of the potatoes and spoon over the other half of the sauce.

Salmon Fishcakes

Serves 4

Ingredients: -

450g cooked mashed sweet potatoes

300g cooked salmon – flaked

2 tbsp. gherkins – chopped

2 tbsp. capers

½ tsp. English mustard

Flour for dusting

1 egg – beaten

85g wholemeal breadcrumbs

Heat the oven to 200C / gas 6

Mix together the mashed potato, fish, gherkins, capers and mustard.

Shape into 4 rounds and lightly dust with flour, cover with Clingfilm and leave in the fridge for 30 minutes.

Dip each cake into the beaten egg and coat in the breadcrumbs.

Place the cakes in a baking tray, drizzle with a little oil and cook for 20 minutes.

Oranges

Oranges are packed with vitamin C. Vitamin C prevents inflammation and strengthens the collagen in your skin. Strengthened collagen helps to smooth the appearance of cellulite and reducing inflammation will lessen the excess weight around a cellulite prone area, in turn decreasing the severity of cellulite. Oranges also contain methoxylated bioflavonoids which help improve the blood circulation and correct imbalances in cells that may lead to cellulite.

Hawaiian Sunset

Serves 2

Ingredients: -
1 papaya – peeled and deseeded
2 passion fruit – flesh scooped out
4 oranges – peeled

Place all the ingredients into a blender and blend until smooth.

Orange, Carrot and Avocado Salad

Serves: - 4

Ingredients: -

2 oranges – peel and cut into segments

1 orange – zest and juice

3 carrots – halved lengthways and sliced with a potato peeler

70g rocket

2 avocados – peeled, stoned and sliced

1 tbsp. extra virgin olive oil

Place the orange segments, carrot strips and avocado slices into a bowl, and gently stir through the rocket.

Whisk together the orange juice, zest and oil, toss through the salad and serve.

Rose Hips

Rose hips can be made into a syrup and drunk as a winter tonic or drunk as a tea. Rose hips have been recognised for their qualities for centuries, in herbal lore the rose is believed to be good for the skin and soul. Amongst rose hips many health benefits they aid blood circulation, flush out excess toxins and hydrate the skin.

Rosemary

Rosemary is believed to improve the body's digestion of fats keeping wastes from building up, including cellulite deposits.

Rosemary and Maple Syrup Parsnips

Serves 4

Ingredients: -
500g parsnips – peeled and quartered lengthways
4 tbsp. olive oil
2 tbsp. chopped rosemary – only use the leaves
3 tbsp. maple syrup

Heat the oven to 200C / gas 6.
Toss the parsnips in the oil and rosemary and season with salt and pepper.
Place the parsnips into a roasting try and roast for 30 minutes, drizzle with the maple syrup and roast for a further 15 minutes until golden and sticky.

Seeds

Flaxseeds, sesame seeds, pumpkin seeds and the oil derived from them are all good sources of vitamin E which is essential for healthy skin and magnesium, iron protein and fibre. Seeds help maintain healthy skin, regulate your appetite and lower your cholesterol. Seeds are high in protein and healthy fats, they have one of the lowers GI values of all foods, which means that they help maintain steady blood sugar levels which results in balanced energy levels with minimal fat storage.

Spinach

Low calorie spinach will not only help you improve your skin but it will also help you lose weight. Spinach is high in vitamin A, which aids the production of collagen in the skin helping to reduce the appearance of cellulite. Collagen is a protein that helps to strengthen, smooth and plump up the skin.

Fresh Spinach Risotto
Serves 2

Ingredients: -
1 onion – finely chopped
3 tbsp. olive oil
200g mixed wild rice
400ml vegetable stock
250g spinach leaves
50g freshly grated parmesan

Cook the rice as per the packet instructions adding a stock cube to the rice water as it comes to the boil. When cooked drain.

Heat the olive oil in a separate pan and gently fry the onion until soft, add the cooked wild rice to the onions and mix. Place the spinach into a blender and blend until it is reduced to pulp, stir it through the rice – add a little more water if it becomes too dry – then stir through the parmesan, season with a little salt and pepper and serve.

Spinach and Fennel Dauphinoise

Serves 4

Ingredients: -

750g Fennel – sliced thinly

450g frozen spinach – defrosted

25g butter

284ml Greek yoghurt if preferred

50g gruyere cheese.

Heat the oven to 160C / gas 4.

Bring a pan of water to the boil and add the sliced fennel and boil for 2 minutes, drain and run under cold water, drain thoroughly.

Squeeze all the liquid from the spinach and season lightly.

Grease a baking dish.

Layer 1/3 of the fennel slices over the base of a gratin dish.

Dot with a third of the butter and season with salt and pepper.

Spread over 1/3 of the spinach and top with 1/3 of the yoghurt.

Repeat the layers again and then finish with a layer of fennel, pour over the last of the yoghurt and top with the grated gruyere cheese and dot with the remaining butter.

Bake for 1 – 1 ¼ hours until the fennel is tender, and the cheese is golden brown.

Spinach and Ricotta Soup

Serves: - 4

Ingredients: -

3 tbsp. olive oil

3 white onions – peeled and chopped

Sea salt, black pepper

150ml white wine

1 ltr. Vegetable stock

80g flat leaf parsley

A squeeze of lemon juice

4 tbsp. ricotta

Heat the oil in a large sauce pan over a medium to low heat, add the onions, scatter over a teaspoon of salt and sweat for 15 – 20 minutes until soft.

Add the wine, turn the heat up and cook to reduce the liquid by half. Pour in the stock, bring to the boil, then add the spinach and half the parsley.

Bring back to the boil, cover and cook over a low heat for 10 minutes. Add the remaining parsley then pour the soup into a blender and blend until smooth.

Just before serving, re heat the soup, season with salt and pepper, add the squeeze of lemon juice and stir in the ricotta.

Bulghar and Spinach Fritters

Serves: - 4

Ingredients: -
100g bulghar wheat

250g spinach

1 onion – finely chopped

1 garlic clove – crushed

85g fresh wholemeal breadcrumbs

1 egg – beaten

1 tbsp. olive oil

Boil the bulghar wheat for about 5 minutes - until tender, drain and place in a bowl.

Put the spinach into a colander and pour over boiling water from the kettle to wilt it. Cool under running water, squeeze out the liquid, chop and add it to the bulghar with the onion, garlic and breadcrumbs. Season well.

Place half the mix into a blender and blend until it forms a thick paste. Return it to the other half of the mix and combine along with the beaten egg. Mix together, then shape into 8 patties, chill for 30 minutes or until ready to cook.

Heat the oil in a frying pan and fry the patties until crisp on both sides. Serve with a salsa or relish.

Spinach and Lentil Dhal

Serves: - 4

Ingredients: -

300g sweet potatoes – peeled and cut into cubes

250g red lentils

1 tsp. ground turmeric

1 ltr. Hot vegetable stock

1 tsp. ground cumin

½ tsp. ground coriander

2 tbsp. olive oil

1 onion – sliced

3 garlic cloves – crushed

1 tsp. garam masala

100g bag baby spinach

Coriander – chopped – to decorate

Place the sweet potato cubes into a large pan with the lentils, turmeric and stock. Bring to the boil and then simmer, uncovered for 20 minutes, stirring occasionally.

Heat the oil in a pan and fry the onions gently until soft, stir in the garlic, garam masala and the spices – cook for a further 2 minutes.

Stir the spiced onion into the lentils and over a low heat add the spinach, a handful at a time, stirring until wilted. Season well.

Serve with natural yoghurt and chopped coriander

Tomatoes

Tomatoes vibrant red colour comes from lycopene which stimulates the circulatory system and reduces fluid retention. Tomatoes are also rich in vitamin C which helps to keep the skin firm and tout by aiding the production of collagen.

Tomato and Rice Soup

Serves 4

Ingredients: -

400g tin of chopped tomatoes

1 tbsp. tomato puree

1 litre vegetable stock

140g mixed basmati and wild rice

2 tsp. olive oil

1 red onion – chopped

1 carrot – peeled and chopped

1 celery stick – sliced

2 tbsp. balsamic vinegar

1 tbsp. brown sugar

15g flat leaf parsley – chopped

Heat the oil in a large pan and cook the onion, carrots and celery until soft, add the sugar and vinegar and cook for a further minute before adding the tomato puree.

Add the chopped tomatoes, vegetable stock and rice. Cover and simmer for 20 minutes until the rice is cooked.

Season with salt and pepper and a sprinkling of chopped parsley.

Tomato Salad

Serves 4

Ingredients

Handful of parsley – roughly chopped

4 tbsp. extra virgin olive oil

1 tbsp lemon juice

6 anchovy fillets in olive oil – drained

220g tinned tuna – in olive oil – drained

5 tbsp – mayonnaise

1 garlic clove – crushed

3 tbsp. capers

750g mixed tomatoes

. Place the olive oil and parsley into a blender and blend. Add the lemon juice, anchovies, mayonnaise, garlic and 1 tbsp capers to the food processor and blend until smooth.

Roughly chop some of the tomatoes and slice the others, arrange on a serving platter, season with salt and pepper, flake over the drained tuna and pour over the dressing.

Serve with the remaining capers and the parsley oil.

Tomato Risotto

Serves: - 4

Ingredients: -

250ml tomato juice

1 ltre. Vegetable stock

2 tbsp. olive oil

1 medium red onion – finely chopped

1 garlic clove – crushed

6 sun – dried tomatoes in oil – drained and sliced

4 plum tomatoes – chopped

350g risotto rice

25g basil leaves

Pour the tomato juice and vegetable stock into a large pan and bring to a gentle simmer.

Heat the oil in a separate pan, add the onions and garlic and cook until soft.

Stir in the rice and coat it in the oil, then add a ladle of the hot stock. Cook over a low heat and keep stirring until the liquid has been absorbed. Continue until almost all of the stock has been added – approximately 20 minutes.

Add the tomatoes and basil along with the remaining stock and continuing to stir, cook until the rice is tender and the stock has been absorbed.

Season and decorate with chopped herbs and a sprinkling of grated parmesan before serving.

Mediterranean Stuffed Tomatoes.

This also works well with small courgettes and marrows

Serves 4

Ingredients

8 large beef tomatoes

4 tbsp olive oil

1 large onion, finely chopped

85g pine nuts

wholemeal breadcrumbs – made from 4 slices of brown bread

1 garlic cloves

50g black olives – finely chopped

1 tbsp capers

3 tbsp chopped parsley

100g soft goats cheese

. Heat the oven to 190C/ gas 5.

. Cut the tops off the tomatoes and scoop out the pulp and seeds.

. pour 3 tbsp of olive oil into a pan add the garlic and onions and fry for about 5 minutes until lightly coloured.

. Add the pine nuts and breadcrumbs and stir to coat in the oil and continue to cook for about 10 minutes until the nuts and breadcrumbs are nicely toasted.

. Remove from the heat and add the olives, flesh of the tomatoes, capers and parsley and season with salt and pepper.

. Place the scooped-out tomatoes into an oven proof dish, place a slice of goat's cheese into the bottom of each tomato and fill with the mixture.

. Drizzle over the last teaspoon of olive oil and bake for 35 – 40 minutes until the tomatoes are tender and the filling is crispy.

Serve warm

.

Turmeric

Like Cayenne pepper, turmeric can help getting rid of cellulite. Turmeric is known for its high levels of antioxidants, it stimulates the circulation, reduces swelling and helps to flush out toxins from the body.

Lentil Dhal
Serves 4

Ingredients: -
300g red lentils
¾ tsp. turmeric
75g fresh ginger
4 tbsp. sunflower oil
1 tsp. cumin seeds
¾ tsp. chilli flakes
1 large onion – finely chopped
6 garlic cloves – crushed
¾ tsp. garam masala
2 tomatoes – cut into wedges
2 tbsp. chopped coriander

Place the lentils in a large pan with the turmeric and 1.5 litres of water. Cut the ginger in half and add 1 half to the pan.

Simmer the lentils for about 1 ½ hours until soft and tender, remove the ginger.

Heat the oil in a pan and add the cumin seeds and chilli flakes, cook gently for about 30 seconds until they give off a spicy aroma. Add the onion to the pan and continue cooking until tender.

Chop the other half of the ginger, finely and add it to the pan with the crushed garlic – cook for a further 2 minutes. Add the garam masala and tomatoes and cook for another minute before pouring the mixture into the cooked lentils.

Stir in the chopped coriander and season before serving.

Watermelon

Watermelon contains the antioxidant lycopene which is where it gets its wonderful colour from. Lycopene helps to improve blood circulation which can over time help to smooth out cellulite.

Crimson Sunset
Serves 4

Ingredients: -
¼ small watermelon – seeds removed
125g raspberries
1 orange – juiced

Place all the ingredients into a blender and blend until smooth.

Wholegrains

Whole grain cereals, oats, rye, barley, wheat, buckwheat, quinoa, millet and brown rice are all a source of slow release energy helping us to feel fuller for longer. Whole grains keep the body's blood sugar levels balanced, preventing energy spikes which lead to cravings for sugary foods – sugary foods cause cellulite.

Whole grains are also high in antioxidants which help the body to flush out toxins which can lead to cellulite.

Printed in Great Britain
by Amazon